The l  For
Medical Instructors

The Pocket Guide to Teaching For Medical Instructors

Advanced Life Support Group

Edited by

KEVIN MACKWAY-JONES
AND
MIKE WALKER

in collaboration with the Resuscitation Council (UK)

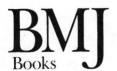

© BMJ Books 1999
BMJ Books is an imprint of the BMJ Publishing Group

First published in 1998
by BMJ Books, BMA House, Tavistock Square,
London WC1H 9JR
Reprinted 1999
Reprinted 2000 (twice)
Reprinted 2001 (twice)

British Library Cataloguing in Publication Data

A catalogue record for this book is available from the
British Library

ISBN: 0–7279–1380–8

Typeset by Apek Typesetters, Nailsea, Bristol
Printed and bound in Great Britain by J. W. Arrowsmith Ltd, Bristol

Contents

Working Group

Bob Bingham
Vice Chairman, Resuscitation Council (UK)

Breege Byrne
Coordinator, Resuscitation Council (UK)

Mike Davis
PALS Educator, Advanced Life Support Group

Sara Harris
Instructor Course Coordinator, Resuscitation Council (UK)

Kevin Mackway-Jones
Executive Director, Advanced Life Support Group

Sheila Simpson
Resuscitation Training Officer, Great Ormond Street

Susan Wieteska
International Coordinator, Advanced Life Support Group

Mike Walker
Educator, Resuscitation Council (UK)

Contributors

Mike Davis
Lecturer in Education, University of Manchester

Peter Driscoll
Senior Lecturer in Emergency Medicine, University of Manchester

Carl Gwinnutt
Consultant Anaesthetist, Hope Hospital, Salford

Lynn Jones
Lecturer in Education, University of Manchester

Kevin Mackway-Jones
Consultant Emergency Physician, Manchester Royal Infirmary

Mike Walker
Senior Lecturer in Medical Education, Imperial College, London

Terence Wardle
Consultant Physician, Countess of Chester Hospital, Chester

Preface

This short guide is presented in two parts. Part One begins by introducing the basic principles underlying teaching and then goes on to deal in more detail with a number of modes of teaching found on Advanced Life Support courses. Lectures, skill stations, scenarios, workshops and discussions are dealt with here. In each case practical guidance is given to help the reader to become a more effective teacher.

Part Two covers many of the same areas again, but this time giving more background information, and describing some more advanced instructional skills. It deals with the nature of adult learning, the four domains of learning, the learning process, questions and answers, role play, mentoring, and problems with workshops and discussions. Each topic is presented as a short section which can be sampled to help with specific issues.

The guide is intended as an aid to reflection: something which you can, and hopefully will, consult on many occasions before, during, and after teaching your courses. It does not contain all the answers, but it will at least provide an alternative voice, something to argue with and something against which you can test your experiences. This guide does not attempt to provide a blueprint for teaching, rather it gives advice about the basics which, once mastered, will be adapted to your personality and creativity. In the end, of course, it is what works for you that matters.

In the long run it does not matter greatly whether you read this guide before or after a course (although most courses will require you to read beforehand). Knowledge and skill as a teacher build up gradually, provided you are able to reflect upon your teaching experiences and continue to learn.

Good luck with your teaching.

Kevin Mackway-Jones
Mike Walker

Acknowledgments

A great many people have put a lot of hard work into the production of this book, and the accompanying Generic Instructor Course. The editors would like to thank all the contributors for their efforts. Thanks are due to Duncan Harris in particular for his efforts in guiding the early developments.

We are greatly indebted to Helen Carruthers for producing the excellent line drawings that illustrate the text.

Finally, we would like to thank, in advance, those of you who will attend the Generic Instructor Course; no doubt, you will have much constructive criticism to offer.

PART ONE

BASIC PRINCIPLES

1 Introduction

This first chapter sets out the basic principles of teaching which will be used throughout the guide. These principles can be used to plan and deliver all forms of teaching, whether lectures, discussions, workshops, or skill stations.

Teaching may be defined as a **planned experience which brings about a change in behaviour.** The important words here are "planned" and "change in behaviour". We all learn from experience, but teaching involves a planned intention to bring about the learning of specified material which will result in a desired form of behaviour.

There are always four elements to consider:

- **Environment**
- **Set**
- **Dialogue**
- **Closure**

These are discussed in more detail below.

Environment

The teaching environment is an integral part of the teaching process. All aspects of the environment should be considered. These include the heating, the lighting, the ventilation, the acoustics, and the arrangement of the furniture.

The environment can radically affect how a teaching session is conducted and how it will be interpreted by the learners. For example, serried rows of chairs restrict participation, whereas a circle implies that everyone is expected to contribute. Suboptimal heating and lighting can undermine a teaching session which has otherwise been meticulous in its preparation. Students who cannot hear the instructor or see the demonstration will have no teaching at all.

The environment must, then, be conducive to the learning that has been planned.

Set

This is the first part of the instructor/learner contact and, as such, is a key part of any teaching session. The set must establish the following:

- Mood
- Motivation
- Objectives
- Roles

Set takes place in the first few minutes of any session. It is during this time that the instructor will establish the **mood** suggested by the environment and enhance the learners' **motivation** by demonstrating the usefulness of the content for them. During set, the **objectives** will be stated and the learner's and instructor's **roles** will be made clear, for example, the learners should be told whether they are to be active or passive, ask questions or participate in other ways.

Set prepares the teaching group for learning.

Dialogue

This is the main part of the planned experience, and involves an interaction between learner and teacher that brings about the planned change in behaviour.

There are many ways of conducting the dialogue – the instructor may lecture throughout, may facilitate a candidate discussion or may use some combination of these. Whatever technique is used, the instructor must ensure that the content is available to the learner in a clear and logical form, and at a level which can be understood.

Checking whether the ideas have been understood usually involves questions and answers in one form or another. Giving an appropriate response to the learner's question or comment – a response that promotes learning – is the essence of dialogue.

Closure

The final part of the teaching session should be the closure. A teaching session which does not end clearly but just peters out not only has an unsatisfactory feel about it, but may also leave unanswered questions in the student's mind. A good closure has three parts:

- Questions
- Summary
- Termination

A period for questions from the students allows any remaining problems to be aired and dealt with. A concise summary pulls together the key points of the session and can relate them to other areas. Finally, the termination ends the session. The latter can be achieved in a variety of ways. The most obvious is direct verbal instruction linked with a break in eye contact and a physical move away from the class.

In the sections which follow you will find that each mode of teaching is broken down into the four constituent phases – environment, set, dialogue and closure – discussed above.

2 Lectures

This chapter is concerned with lecturing skills. After reading it you should:

- **understand** the range of lecturing techniques
- **be aware** of the variety of visual aids available
- **be able** to prepare a lecture

Environment

The layout of the teaching area is central to the nature of the lecture. A room set out in rows conveys a more formal atmosphere and may be more conducive to conveying information, whereas a room set out with chairs in a semi-circle suggests a more interactive approach. Similarly, the presence of desks will suggest to candidates that notes should be taken.

In order to control the environment, instructors need to arrive at the teaching venue in advance. The instructor must make decisions based on the needs of both candidates and lecturer and should consider audio visual presentation and the need to maintain interest.

The level of lighting and heating during the lecture must be controlled. Bright lighting will encourage learners to stay awake and enables them to take as many notes as they like; a darkened room not only encourages quite the opposite, but also makes it more difficult to see the audience and to maintain eye contact. At worst, a warm, stuffy room used after lunch encourages sleeping and may not be conducive to any learning at all.

Modern lecture facilities may contain a number of aids for the lecturer, including back projection, amplification (including loop induction for the hard of hearing), video and much else. It is essential that the technical aspects of this equipment are mastered. Inability to operate a slide projector, laser pointer, or the ambient light circuit gives the learners the impression that the lecturer has failed to prepare properly; they may also conclude from this that the content of the lecture is also suspect.

Set

In many situations learners will have received written material prior to attending for instruction. As most adult learners are highly motivated to achieve the standard required, they will probably have read these materials in detail. They may therefore consider lectures as being optional since they know that they have acquired the basic knowledge already. It is essential that lecturers overcome this feeling during the set, and involve all the candidates in the lecture. The set must be established in terms of:

• Mood
• Motivation
• Objectives
• Roles

The environmental changes made prior to the learners' arrival help set the mood. Instructors can reinforce this by varying tone of voice, actions, and pace of presentation. The learners' motivation can be increased by identifying the usefulness of the material, typically by relating the content to the learners' experience.

A clear statement of the learning objectives of each session is necessary. It is important that learners are told exactly what it is that they will be expected to know or be able to do by the end of the session and how this will link with other parts of the course.

The learners' role should be explicitly stated so that they are clear about how they will participate in the teaching session. They need to know if they should be silent recipients, contribute when asked, or be the main participants. The message can usually be got over using a mixture of simple statements and body language.

Dialogue

Proper planning is necessary to ensure that lectures have a clear purpose and line of development, and that they link coherently with other areas of learning. In order to have credibility with the learners, instructors must demonstrate expertise in relation to the content of their lecture.

Content

The broad content of lectures will often be prescribed by a curriculum, by slide sets provided or by other guidelines. However, there is always scope for individual lecturers to select, prioritise or otherwise emphasise elements of the content. Such selection will be guided by a knowledge of the particular audience for whom the lecture is being prepared. The composition of the audience, their backgrounds, working environment and experience will guide the lecturer in preparing a lecture which will provide optimum learning for this particular audience.

Delivery

Many lecturers, particularly those new to lecturing, write out a complete script of everything they will say. Reading a script however is really a last resort, and notes are often sufficient for familiar material. These can usually be transferred to slides or overhead projector acetates. The list of 3, 4 or 5 points (seldom any more) on the slide acts both as an *aide-mémoire* for the lecturer and as a structure for the audience. It may be useful for the new lecturer to summarise the main points on one page. This is best committed to memory.

Lecturers preparing new material may find it helpful to verbally rehearse the content, silently or out loud. This increases familiarity with the content and highlights transitions that are not smooth or points that are unclear. It also gives an indication of the time that the session will take.

There are a number of ways of delivering the dialogue. These may be summarised as:

- Talking
- Talking and writing
- Questions and answers
- Audience activities
- Demonstrations

Talking

This is the classical method of lecture delivery and may be used with or without audio visual aids. The lecturer stands in front of the learners and talks to them about the subject matter. Talking can be combined with the use of slides (often provided on courses) or with pre-prepared overhead acetates or other visual aids.

From an audience perspective this can easily become a passive experience. Lecturers must ensure that they involve the audience in the presentation if they are to maintain attention. Attention can also be increased simply by moving around the room, establishing eye contact, and by directly talking to different sections of the audience. Using techniques such as these, a lecturer can establish the notion that each learner is being addressed.

Talking and writing

This method has been called "chalk and talk". It does not actually matter whether the writing is done on a blackboard with chalk, on a whiteboard or a flipchart with a pen, or on a blank acetate. The concept is the same. The lecturer has a structure for the session and summarises key points by writing them down so that the class can see them. These can be used as an *aide-mémoire* following discussion, or as a guide for student note taking. These visual media may also be used for drawing diagrams or pictures to illustrate the points being made. Visual representation is a powerful aid to learning and the drawing of images creates intense audience interest, even where the image itself is fairly primitive. It is not necessary to be an "artist" to draw visual representations that will enhance learning very effectively.

Questions and answers

Many methods incorporate question and answer techniques. These techniques are a useful way to engage learners in an issue, or to set up a problem that groups will be motivated to explore. They also provide a way of evaluating participants' understanding of the topics thus far.

Clear straightforward questions which allow anyone to respond, are generally better than complex questions that are directed towards one person.

Time should be given for people to reflect and frame an answer; this may involve a short silence. If one learner is still unable to answer, then the question may be rephrased if it lacked clarity, additional cues to respond can be given, or another candidate can be directly approached.

It is important to receive answers positively. For one thing, warm verbal and non-verbal signals will encourage people to speak and to feel that their contribution is valued, and for another, the rest of the audience will feel encouraged to participate once they feel it is safe to do so. It is not always best to be evaluative ("that's right" or "no"), following an answer. Instead, the rest of the group can be encouraged to take on the discussion or to add alternative views ("How do the rest of you feel about that?"). Strategies generally associated with counselling skills can be useful ways of processing responses – accepting, clarifying, reframing, etc. Often this involves paraphrasing, which has the additional function of repeating the point for those who did not hear it or reinforcing it without direct repetition. Total translating ("So what you are really saying is . . .") followed by a statement which bears no relation to the candidate's original should be avoided since it is patronising.

When the question and answer method of delivery is used in a lecture, the instructor uses the candidates' replies to a series of questions to take the candidates in a controlled way through the subject matter. Actually, the question and answer method is one of the most difficult methods to get right and it will be reconsidered in Part Two.

Audience activities

Brainstorming

Brainstorming generates lots of ideas really quickly. People are asked to call out any answers they have to a question or suggestions or issues raised by a topic. All ideas should be written up on a board or flip chart. It is important that *everything* is written up, and nothing is processed at this stage (i.e. no feedback is given, responses are just noted). No contributions are criticised or minimised, as the idea is to encourage maximum participation at speed.

This is the easy part of brainstorming and if it is left at this point ("Well that *is* an interesting list of words!") it has little value. The value comes in the analysis of the answers. Thus the lecturer has to be able to detect and show patterns in the seemingly random answers and to demonstrate that these patterns hold significant insights.

For example, among the dozen or so ideas recorded during a brainstorming session on how adults learn are the following:

ask questions
discuss
investigate
share with others
participate
consult

The lecturer would recognise, here, that each of these words implies an active component from which it could be argued that adults prefer to learn in an active rather than a passive mode.

Buzz groups

Pairs or small groups of individuals may be given a question or an issue to discuss for a few minutes. This technique provides a break during a lecture and also generates energy and increases participation. When the level of noise reduces or an appropriate amount of time has elapsed, feedback can be taken on the key issues. This should be done rapidly and informally, rather than as a question and answer session or discussion group feedback. Here again, it is the use made of the answers provided from buzz groups that is important – the way in which the answers are incorporated and made an integral part of the lecture.

Demonstrations

Demonstrations with apparatus clearly have a separate and special place on many practical courses.

There may be times when talking about a practical procedure can only provide a static view even when the talk is augmented by a slide. In such circumstances a dynamic element can be introduced by placing a model on an overhead projector and showing the procedure in silhouette.

Showing actual apparatus always increases interest but can be distracting. All demonstration materials should be retrieved before the lecture is continued. The apparatus can be made available for further inspection at the end of the session.

Audio visual aids

Each method of delivery can be combined with the use of various audio visual aids. These include:

11

- Slide projector
- Overhead projector
- Computer and projector
- Blackboard/whiteboard
- Flip chart
- Apparatus

Slides

Many instructors are extremely familiar with the use of slides, and many courses have set slides as a key teaching aid. In general, slide sets have been constructed to lend themselves to the set, dialogue, closure paradigm; many courses include optional slides which can be used for question and answer sessions. Often, picture slides are included both to break up the text and to illustrate particular points.

Lecturers may wish to construct their own slide sets, and supplement the slide sets provided for lectures that they are allocated to teach. These additional slides may be text slides, or picture slides.

Text slides When constructing text slides, certain rules should be followed and these are summarised below. There should be:

- a maximum 7 lines in height
- a maximum 7 words in width
- a maximum 5 words in the title
- simple text or diagrams

A number of slides are shown in Figure 2.1.

In general, text slides are used as an *aide-mémoire* both for the lecturer and the students.

Picture slides Picture slides are always interesting. Lecturers must be careful to ensure that the picture slides they select have direct relevance to that part of the lecture in which they are going to be used. It is tempting to show an "interesting" picture which does not have direct relevance. It is also tempting to show too many pictures. Lecturers should always remember that they have objectives, and all slides should be there with the aim of achieving the objectives of the teaching session.

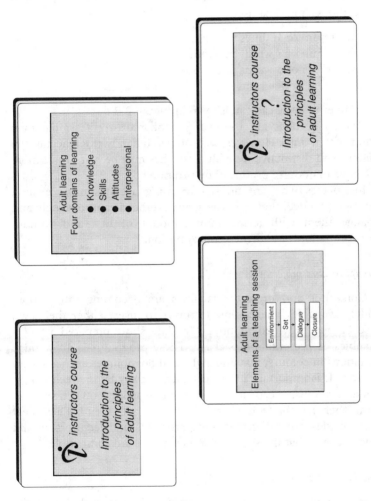

Figure 2.1   Example of a number of slides

Overheads

Acetate sheets on an overhead projector can either be used as a talk and write aid, or can be pre-prepared. In the latter case exactly the same general comments apply as those given for slides. Since the shape of overheads is slightly different, the following preparation guides should be used:

• a maximum of 10 lines in height
• a maximum of 7 words in width
• a maximum of 5 words in the title
• simple text or diagrams

A number of overheads are shown in Figure 2.2.

Printed acetates are thought to look more professional than handwritten ones. However, well-prepared handwritten acetates in colour with distinctive individual touches may be just, if not more effective than those produced by computer.

Instructors who are unused to using acetates must ensure, through practice, that they can place overheads appropriately and change them with a minimum amount of fuss and without disrupting flow or audience concentration.

Computer and projector

Computer and projector facilities are becoming much more widely available. These allow lecturers to insert either their own disc or one provided to project a slide show prepared using a graphics or presentation package. These programmes allow huge variations in colours, text and style, and possibilities are seemingly endless. It is important not to get carried away by the technology. Lecturers must keep in mind their teaching objectives and remember that the technology is a means, not an end. These new technologies can bring their own problems and lecturers should always check that the software and hardware are compatible.

Blackboards/whiteboards

In general blackboards and whiteboards are used during the "talk and write" form of teaching. Writing on a vertical surface needs practice and writing **legibly** on a vertical surface needs more practice still. It is essential that this skill is mastered before these aids are used, and that the lecturer then ensures that the writing can be read from the back as well as the front of the room. Carrying

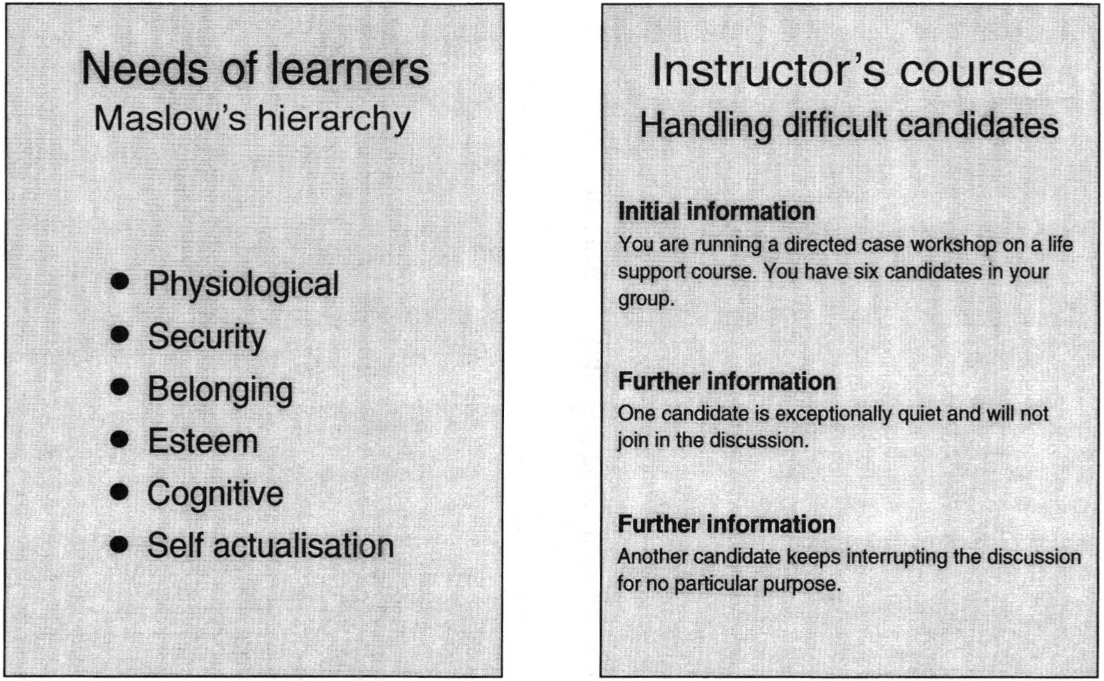

Needs of learners
Maslow's hierarchy

- Physiological
- Security
- Belonging
- Esteem
- Cognitive
- Self actualisation

Instructor's course
Handling difficult candidates

Initial information
You are running a directed case workshop on a life support course. You have six candidates in your group.

Further information
One candidate is exceptionally quiet and will not join in the discussion.

Further information
Another candidate keeps interrupting the discussion for no particular purpose.

Figure 2.2   Example of a number of overheads

15

spare chalk or a whiteboard pen prevents the disruption of a session due to a lack of basic equipment.

Flip chart

Much of what has been said about blackboards and whiteboards also applies to flip charts. The advantage of the flip chart over the whiteboard is that it is easy to go back to previous sheets, and therefore to illustrate previous ideas. Flip charts should not be used as a scribbling pad for the instructor – this will totally confuse the learners.

Sheets of flipchart paper may be used by candidates to summarise small group discussions during feedback at the end of an activity.

Closure

Closure should include the following elements:

- Questions
- Summary
- Termination

It is essential that time is left at the end of the lecture for candidates to ask questions. All questions should be answered if possible, but answers need to be given within the time limits. If it would be too complex, contentious, or irrelevant to answer a question during the lecture then the learner should be given the opportunity to meet with an instructor later to discuss the point raised. During courses there are usually other instructors at the back of the lecture room, and the lecturer may wish to involve these teachers in the answering of questions as well.

A summary should be given at the end of each lecture session. This should include the key points, and may also include summaries of questions and contentious issues.

Once the summary has been given, it is important to ensure that there is a clear termination. This may be physical, such as the lecturer leaving the room, or verbal such as a handover to another lecturer, or may take the form of a directive to go to another area for another teaching session.

Lecture checklist

Environment

- Fix layout
- Check lighting
- Adjust heating/ventilation
- Check equipment

Set

- Set mood
- Establish usefulness/identify relevance
- State learning objectives
- Clarify learner and teacher roles

Dialogue

- Organise content in clear logical sequence
- Coordinate content with appropriate visual aids
- Ensure voice projection
- Address the audience and ensure eye contact
- Draw from personal and audience experience to illustrate and apply points
- Demonstrate enthusiasm for the topic and for teaching
- Use humour appropriately
- Ask appropriate questions
- Respond positively to answers
- Use answers
- Summarise main points at intervals
- Establish links with other teaching sessions

Closure

- Ask for questions or comments
- Return to learning objectives and summarise
- Terminate session

Example lecture plan

Environment

Layout

Check seating adequate
Check visibility from seats
Check lighting
Adjust heating/ventilation

Equipment

Check audio visual equipment function
Test all controls

Equipment list

Slides
Slide projector
Slide projector remote control
Laser pointer
Other aids

Set

Introduce yourself to the audience
Explain the usefulness and relevance of the topic:

> "I am going to introduce you to one of the most important topics of the course . . ."

State the learning objectives:

> "By the end of the session you should be able to understand the need for basic airway positioning and clearing and where necessary the use of advanced airway adjuncts."

Clarify the roles of learner and teacher:

> "The lecture will take about half an hour but there will be times when I will want to ask you questions and also times when I will pause for you to ask me questions. Is that clear?"

Dialogue

Example of slide list

One Day PLS Course

LECTURE 4: AIRWAY & VENTILATION

No.	Label	Description
1	PLSAM01	Title Airway & Ventilation
2	APLSAM02	Airway Manoeuvres
3	APLSAM03	Airway – basic manoeuvres 1
4	APLSAM04	Airway – basic manoeuvres 2
5	APLSAM05	Picture – wall-mounted suction
6	APLSAM06	Airway Adjuncts
7	APLSAM07	Airway Adjuncts Oropharyngeal
8	APLSAM08	Picture – paediatric O/P airways
9	APLSAM09	Picture – O/P airway in situ
10	APLSAM10	Airway Adjuncts Nasopharyngeal
11	APLSAM11	Airway Adjuncts ETT selection
12	APLSAM12	Picture – paediatric endotracheal tubes
13	APLSAM13	Intubation – before starting
14	APLSAM14	Intubation equipment
15	APLSAM15	Picture – laryngoscopes
16	APLSAM16	Intubation – after insertion
17	APLSAM17	Oxygen and Intubation
18	APLSAM18	Intubation – complications
19	APLSAM24	Ventilation – BLS revision
20	APLSAM25	Oxygen Delivery – methods
21	APLSAM26	O_2 – highest possible concentration
22	PLSAM27	Ventilation – methods list
23	APLSAM28	Picture – self-inflating bag
24	APLSAM29	Picture – open-ended bag
25	APLSAM30	Ventilation – face mask properties
26	PLSAM33	Question Airway and Ventilation
27	APLSAM34	A&V – Summary 1
28	PLSAM35	A&V – Summary 2

Closure

Ask if there are any questions
Summarise:

> "In this session we have covered the following . . ."

Terminate the session

3 Skills teaching

This chapter is concerned with the teaching of psychomotor skills. After reading it you should:

- **understand** the four-stage procedure for teaching skills
- **be aware** of the problems of time management in skills teaching
- **be able** to prepare a skills teaching session

The teaching of skills usually takes place in small groups. Such teaching situations are commonly referred to as skill stations. From the learner's perspective skill stations are a combination of psychomotor skill acquisition and a discussion. The latter enables problems to be expressed and conflicts with previous teaching to be solved; it also enables teachers to place skills in context.

Students being taught psychomotor skills often come from different backgrounds, with varying experience and requirements. These differences are more apparent in skills teaching than in any other form of teaching. Instructors should make an effort to get to know the candidates' backgrounds and take this into account.

Feedback is particularly important to the learners and this is especially so during the dialogue. Positive feedback in context helps ensure retention of accurate skill performance, while constructively phrased correction helps to abolish incorrect actions.

At the end of the teaching session feedback is important to ensure that learners know whether or not they have achieved their goals.

Environment

The adequacy of the environment can make or break the effectiveness of a skill station. Achieving an optimum environment can be complex. Two aspects are considered below – layout and equipment.

Layout

This consists of the location of the skill station and its relationship to its immediate environment. A variety of possible layouts exist. Each station may be in its own room or in a large room with several other stations teaching the same or different skills; individual stations may or may not be screened from one another.

The space allocated for teaching will influence the way in which the session is planned. The aim is always to ensure that the learners are not distracted by "outside" events. This means avoiding setting up the station so that there are distracting activities in the direct line of sight of the students.

As always, temperature is important. This is especially so in skills requiring physical exertions since the room may become stuffy and hot as active bodies generate a lot of heat. Student enthusiasm will wane as discomfort increases.

When setting up the teaching area, the most important thing is that all of the learners can see what is happening. Usually, this is best achieved by allowing access from all sides. If tables are used they may have to be moved away from the wall to achieve this.

Some skills cannot be appreciated unless the learners are orientated correctly and this may mean a change of approach so that they can all observe. If some are required to **do** while others **see**, this means that the learners will need to move around. In these situations it is important to ensure that there are no obstacles to movement; these not only break concentration but also waste time.

Equipment

It is important to construct a mental list of the equipment required to teach the skill effectively. The actual equipment available can then be checked against this list and any deficiencies can be rectified. The easiest way to achieve this is for the instructor to run through the skill beforehand and note any problems.

Whoever provides the equipment, it is always the instructor's responsibility to ensure the effectiveness of the teaching episode.

Thus whatever equipment is provided, teachers must ensure that they are **totally familiar with it.** This means that everything must be tested before the candidates arrive.

Equipment should be presented in a way that recreates a situation as close as possible to that which will be encountered in practice. Laying out pieces in their order of use can be helpful, particularly if the skill is new to several of the candidates. Any apparatus not immediately required for a particular teaching episode should be put on one side to avoid confusion.

Once everything is arranged, covering the equipment with a cloth removes distraction and worry as candidates approach.

Set

For many learners the acquisition of new psychomotor skills is a daunting prospect - this is particularly so if the chance of public failure exists. Therefore it is essential that within the first few moments the set is established and the learner orientated in terms of:

• Mood
• Motivation
• Objectives
• Roles

Motivation to learn new skills is increased when learners understand why the skill is performed and when they perceive that the skill is useful and important. The skill must also be put into context and linked with the rest of the course. The usefulness of the content is emphasised by using either questions such as: "When, in your work, would you use this procedure?", or a direct statement such as, "The purpose of this session is to enable you all to carry out this skill so that . . .".

The candidates must then be given a clear indication of the objectives of the skill station and made aware of what is expected of them by the end of the session, i.e. they must be given goals which are realistic.

Finally, the teacher must identify how the learners are expected to participate in the skill station.

23

Dialogue

This is the main part of the planned experience and requires interaction between the teacher and learners, culminating in individual performance of the skill. A four-part approach is used:

- Instructor demonstrates the skill (without commentary)
- Instructor demonstrates the skill and provides a commentary
- Instructor demonstrates the skill and the learner provides the commentary
- Learner demonstrates the skill and provides the commentary

The constituent parts are discussed in more detail below.

Instructor demonstrates the skill (without commentary)

The purpose of the first stage of the process is to ensure that the learners have a clear picture of what it is they have to learn. They can best achieve this by using their eyes to note every action involved in performing the skill. A commentary at this stage distracts learners – their natural instinct will be to stop watching the demonstration and look at the teacher. A silent demonstration is, therefore, an integral part of the process of psychomotor learning.

It is important to inform the candidates that they are going to see the skill performed at normal speed, and that this is what is expected of them on completion.

Instructor demonstrates the skill and adds a commentary

Once the silent demonstration is completed the skill is demonstrated again. The task is broken down into simple steps, and carried out slowly. Some questions that have formed in the learners' minds will be answered during this second run. Any remaining questions must be answered at the end of this stage.

Instructor demonstrates the skill and the learner adds the commentary

For the third stage a learner is selected to give a commentary as the instructor performs the skill. This stage is a useful part of the learning process because a skill is learned more easily if the learner can describe the entire skill. If a hesitant candidate is talking the skill through it is better to lead with the actions and allow the learner to follow, since this lets them see the manoeuvre again in detail and then describe it. A confident candidate can be allowed to describe the action before it is performed by the instructor.

It is essential that errors made by the learners are corrected immediately. A number of techniques can be used for this. The candidate can be allowed to rethink and compare with the silent run through; the instructor can correct the learner; or, preferably, the problem may be addressed by the group. This stage can be repeated once, twice or even three times using different candidates, depending upon the time available.

Learner demonstrates the skill and adds the commentary

This is the final step and consists of allowing **each** student to perform the skill and describe what they are doing. As this is the guided response level of psychomotor learning, it must be under direct supervision of the instructor. By this stage the student will have seen the skill demonstrated at least three times and heard two descriptions. This reinforcement improves the success rate. By observing each candidate the instructor will also be able to assess whether they have understood and are competent at the skill.

Where time permits, candidates should engage in a fifth stage namely, **practice**.

Closure

This is the process which signals to the learner the end of the session, and, as before, it can be divided into three main elements:

* questions
* summary
* termination

With good planning everybody will have successfully completed the skill. The candidates must again be given the opportunity to ask any remaining questions and voice any difficulties.

The summary should incorporate all the lessons learned, a quick review of the skills, a link to associated knowledge and skills and finally a synthesis of all key issues that arose in the questions.

Termination of the session involves moving the candidates onto the next organised teaching session.

25

Checklist for skill stations

Environment

- Fix layout
- Check lighting
- Adjust heating/ventilation
- Check equipment
- Ensure all students can see clearly
- Ensure adequate movement is possible

Set

- Set mood
- Establish usefulness/identify relevance
- State learning objectives
- Clarify learner and teacher roles

Dialogue

- Describe the four-stage method of teaching (if students are unfamiliar with this)
- Demonstrate the skill – without commentary
- Demonstrate the skill – with commentary
- Demonstrate the skill – with student commentary
- Allow each student to demonstrate the skill and provide a commentary
- Summarise important aspects at intervals
- Relate skill to other aspects of the course
- Enable practice if time allows

Closure

- Invite and answer questions
- Summarise key issues
- Terminate session

Example: A teaching plan for basic life support and management of choking

PRACTICAL SKILL STATION
BASIC LIFE SUPPORT – ADULT

Environment

Layout

Check seating adequate
Check visibility from seats
Check lighting
Adjust heating/ventilation
Check access to manikins

Equipment

Check equipment present and correct
Adult resuscitation manikin with performance assessment monitor × 2
Antibacterial wipes × 2
Tissues (box) × 2

Set

Introduction
Establish usefulness/identify relevance:

> "BLS can save lives."

State learning objectives:

> "By the end of this session you will be able to demonstrate:
> • basic life support for a collapsed patient
> • the management of a choking patient."

Clarify learner and teacher roles:

> "This session will last about half an hour. I will demonstrate each of the skills I expect you to have by the end. I will then talk you through them and let one or more of you talk me through them. Finally, each of you will perform each skill. Please ask any questions at the end of each demonstration."

27

Dialogue

Teach stages of basic life support:

1 SAFE approach
2 Assessment of unconscious level
3 Airway opening manoeuvres
4 Assessment of breathing
5 Assessment of circulation
6 Exhaled air resuscitation
7 Closed chest cardiac compression
   • 1-rescuer CPR
   • 2-rescuer CPR

Teach management of choking skills:

1 Back blows
2 Heimlich manoeuvre
3 Abdominal thrusts

Closure

Ask if there are any questions.
Summarise:

> "In this session we covered the sequence of BLS and the performance of one-person and two-person CPR. We also practised manoeuvres that can be used on patients who are choking."

Terminate the session.

4 Workshops and discussions

This chapter is concerned with the facilitation of workshops and discussions. After reading it you should:

- **understand** the different forms and purposes of workshops, and open or closed discussions
- **be aware** of different techniques for facilitating and controlling workshops and discussions
- **be able** to prepare a workshop session or discussion group

Discussion is effective on its own or as part of a workshop. This is because it reflects the way that adults learn best, in that it is an active means of acquiring information. Participants can make it relevant to their personal needs; furthermore, it provides immediate and usually positive feedback.

Discussion of issues without any stimulus or structure may be fun and may even be informative, but is not necessarily of educational value. In an educational context workshops and discussions are used to reinforce and to expand material that has been presented elsewhere. They also provide an opportunity for learners to develop and articulate their attitudes towards some of the issues and dilemmas inherent in that material.

Workshops

Workshops are usually based on clinical information which is used to guide the discussion. They tend to be task-focused, and require participants to come to some reasoned conclusion concerning the course of action to be taken in the given situation.

29

Closed discussions

Closed discussions resemble workshops in being knowledge-focused. They can be used to impart new knowledge or to revise what should already be known. This kind of discussion is suitable when there is a definitive answer to the questions posed.

Open discussions

Open discussions are used for rather different purposes. They are process-centred – that is, more concerned with what the individuals learn from *participating* in the discussion than with resolving particular issues. The focus for open discussions tends to come from those areas where definitive answers are not available, and from areas where there are ethical dilemmas. Examples include, when to stop resuscitation, whether to allow relatives in the resuscitation room and the issues surrounding "do not resuscitate" orders.

The educational principles described below relate to both workshops and discussions. Where there are important differences between the two, these are indicated.

Environment

As elsewhere, preparation is the key to the successful discussion or workshop. In this context preparation also includes selecting the appropriate topics for discussion and being familiar with the content of any presented material.

The layout of the room is also crucial to the successful running of the session, as it can have a tremendous bearing on the educational effectiveness. Different layouts facilitate different degrees of group interaction. A small, closed circle, is ideal for open discussions. This is illustrated in Figure 4.1. It does not signify a leader and suggests equal opportunities for participation.

A horseshoe with the "chair" person seated at the focus is used for closed discussions – this indicates that discussion will be directed by and through the "chair". The same arrangement may be used for workshops although here the "chair" may also require an OHP to assist in the presentation of case material. This is illustrated in Figure 4.2.

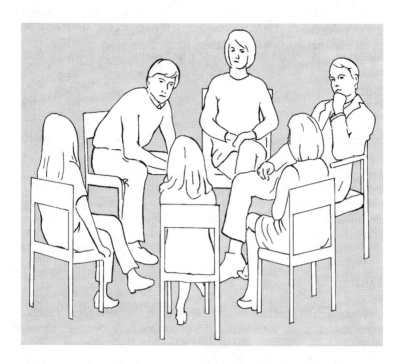

Figure 4.1   Closed circle – ideal for open discussions.

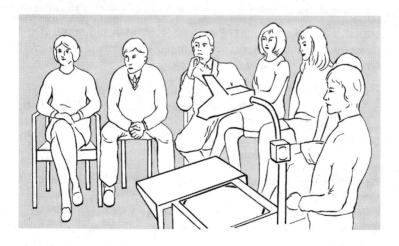

Figure 4.2   Horseshoe arrangement.

An eccentric position for the instructor and projector allows a greater degree of control to be exerted over a candidate, with all contributions made initially to the tutor.

Set

An appropriate mood may be created during the introduction. An informal introduction followed by time spent learning the names of the candidates will help relax the learners. It is important that the general content of the session and its usefulness is outlined. Specific objectives will vary depending on the type of session. In general, they are focused for workshops and closed discussions, but more general for open discussions. They should be stated.

Dialogue

Workshops and closed discussions tend to use a more teacher-centred dialogue, with the majority of questions and comments being directed by and through the tutor. Questions tend to be short, closed and require relatively factual answers. They are, initially at least, of the "what, why, how, when" kind. The tutor in a workshop or closed discussion will tend to put questions to members of the group in turn both to canvas views and to ensure participation. The content of replies can be recorded either on paper, a flip chart or board for use later, as a summary. If it is thought that candidates' answers need developing, then several strategies are available, for instance:

• Asking for individual development: "Why do you say that?"
• Asking for development from the rest of the group: "What do the rest of you think?"
• Asking for development from another individual: "Isn't that what you were saying earlier . . .?"

By using these kinds of questions, the tutor can retain control of the direction and pace of the discussion.

In open discussions the dialogue will be more learner-centred. Thus after the initial "set" the tutor will abdicate the "chair" role by avoiding eye contact with the first member to speak. This means that the speaker has to address remarks to the group or to select another member as a focus. The purpose here is to enable the members to explore their views on difficult and sometimes controversial issues. They should not be allowed to look to the tutor to provide an authoritative answer. Through reflecting on their experiences and testing their views against those of others they should begin to put together a coherent, articulate and professionally defensible position on the difficult issues. This suggests that individual contributions may be longer and more related to what other contributors have to say than is the case in the task-related discussions and workshops. The tutor will need to ensure that all who want to contribute are able to. Questions will tend to encourage reflection, rather than elicit correct answers. Some appropriate questions are shown below.

- "Do you suppose that is really the case?"
- "How does that relate to what you were saying earlier?"
- "Does that fit with your everyday experiences at work?"

Control

Instructors running any type of discussion often see control as an issue. The two types of discussions/workshops use differing control strategies. In workshops and closed discussions the tutor introduces the task and the questioning of group members. Since all answers are then addressed to the tutor he or she retains control. In open discussions the tutor deliberately gives up this initiative in order that group members may talk one to another and may respond without having to go through the "chair". Even so, the tutor may need to retain control either to bring into the debate a member who has made several unsuccessful attempts to contribute or to inhibit someone who is tending to dominate the discussion. Control strategies include:

- Saying the person's name forcefully
- Body language
  - moving forward on your chair
  - putting an arm up (traffic control style) to the person speaking
  - avoiding eye contact

The problems with particular types of learner are discussed in more detail elsewhere (see Handling Difficult Learners, Chapter 11).

Closure

In workshops and closed discussions it is appropriate to ask for any final questions or observations. After open discussions this is less appropriate.

All discussions require a summary. For workshops with directed cases this will almost certainly be known, at least in outline, from the outset. With closed discussions the main points can be listed along with any consensus views on policy or recommendations which the group arrived at. The open discussion is usually more difficult to summarise and a summary may only be possible in the most general terms.

Termination is usually easy to achieve by standing up and moving out of the group.

Discussion checklist

Environment

- Fix layout
- Check lighting
- Adjust heating/ventilation
- Check equipment

Set

- Set mood
- Establish usefulness/identify relevance
- State learning objectives
- Clarify learner and teacher roles

Dialogue

- Introduce topics
- Use appropriate questions
- Draw on students' experiences when trying to make new points
- Respond to diverse opinion or conflict generated by learners
- Use body position and eye movements to involve the group
- Limit personal contribution to enable group participation
- Summarise, or elaborate student responses as a means of reinforcing participation
- Draw out the quiet student and control the over-talkative student
- Use alternative explanations as necessary
- Use supporting material as necessary and in an appropriate way
- Maintain the group's attention throughout the session
- Close each directed case when appropriate

Closure

- Allow students to reflect on their feelings about the content of the session
- Review relevant student concerns during the session
- Review with the group all the major points that have been covered in the session
- Identify the end by appropriate body movement or statement
- Terminate the session

Example of workshop teaching plan

Environment

Layout

Check seating adequate
Arrange appropriate seating plan
Check lighting
Adjust heating/ventilation

Equipmnent

Check audio visual equipment functions
Test all controls
[*Equipment list would appear here as a reminder*]

Set

Introduction
Explain the usefulness and relevance of the topic:

> "For the next 30 minutes, we are going to focus on the
> interpretation of blood gas results. In cardiac arrest manage-
> ment, familiarity with a method of interpretation of these
> results will allow you to quickly assess the situation and
> progress rapidly to further interventions as necessary."

Explain the general content and style of the session:

> "We will be trying out the method we have taught you, by
> looking at four directed cases, all of which will emphasise
> relevant issues. Please ask questions as we go along."

State the specific objectives:

> "On completing this workshop, you should be able to
> interpret arterial blood gas results and discuss appropriate
> therapies."

Dialogue

Acetates of directed cases

Case No.	Diagnosis	Case Aim
1	Hyperventilation	Respiratory alkalosis
2	Likely cause overdose complicating COAD	Mixed respiratory and metabolic acidosis
3	Diabetic ketoacidosis	
4	Acute on chronic respiratory acidosis	Respiratory acidosis
5	Cardiac arrest	Mixed metabolic and respiratory acidosis
6	Milk–alkali syndrome with lactic acidosis	Mixed metabolic alkalosis and metabolic acidosis

Acetates of supporting material

1 Key points
2 Normal blood gas values
3 Method of interpretation of ABGs
4 Algorithm for interpretation of blood gases
5 Modified Flenley diagram
6 Anion gap and acidosis

Closure

Ask if there are any questions
Summarise:

"In this session we have covered the following . . ."

Terminate the session

5 Role play and scenarios

This chapter is concerned with the planning and facilitation of role play and scenario sessions. After reading it you should:

- **understand** the aims of role play and scenario teaching
- **be aware** of how to facilitate role play and scenario sessions
- **be able** to prepare role play and scenario teaching sessions

Role play has not always been a popular method of teaching medicine. It does, however, offer advantages over other teaching and learning techniques in that it offers trainees the opportunity to learn by doing. As the aim of much clinical teaching is to enable trainees to treat patients, any method which approaches the real situation has educational advantages.

Role play involves participants in acting out roles that represent real situations, but allows enough distance for a structured and less intense discussion of the thoughts, feelings and behaviours involved. Role play can give the opportunity to practise a range of responses or situations and therefore can increase the individual's repertoire of behaviours. Students may be anxious about role play and it should be introduced gradually (perhaps with warm-up exercises and once the group know each other). Tutors often make role-playing optional, rather than a compulsory activity. However, role play is important as it allows the student to practise technical and interpersonal skills in a "real" but safe environment.

Five common types of role play are:

- **Improvisation** – students are given a situation to act out using their own responses.
- **Structured roles** – students are given roles with clear instructions as to how the role is to be played.

- **Prepared improvisation** – two or more students are asked to play a role, after the group has decided upon the character of the players and the outcome of the play.
- **Reverse role play** – students play out both sides of a situation or adopt a role other than their normal one in order to gain insight into the perceptions, attitudes and behaviours of others.
- **Exaggerated role play** – clear instructions on exaggerated characters can be less threatening to people who are unused to or uncomfortable with role play. It can also highlight particular problems in interactions in a stereotypical and clear way.

Scenarios are a form of improvised role play in which the management of a patient is enacted using real equipment (made safe), a manikin or suitably briefed and made-up patient model, in a controlled environment. Input from instructors and from patient monitors allows trainees to make decisions and assess situations in a way that mimics life. Scenarios therefore represent a pulling together of knowledge and skills and involve aspects of cognitive, affective, psychomotor, and interpersonal learning.

Debriefing

It is extremely important to debrief after a role play. There are two main aspects to the debrief. The first involves reflection – allowing the participants to say how they felt and what they were feeling during the various stages of the role play. They should be encouraged to share any insights they gained into their own responses or those of others. The second aspect is concerned with returning to normal. Role play can be highly emotionally charged and students can, very quickly, take on the role of a bereaved parent or a distressed spouse which may involve expressing aggression or frustration towards clinical staff. To a certain extent they can "feel" the pain or the anger of those individuals. Care has to be taken to allow them time to talk out their feelings and to be guided back to normality by the instructor.

Environment

The actual nature of this role play or scenario is important when arranging the environment. Role play and scenario teaching are dealt with separately below.

39

Role play

Role plays require planning, and this should address the following issues:

- What are the objectives of the role play and is this the best way of dealing with this topic?
- Is there an atmosphere of trust in which students will feel comfortable acting out their roles?
- Is there enough space to conduct a role play so that all can see, and so that any noise generated will not interfere with other learners?
- Is there enough time to conduct a proper debriefing?
- Are the participants' instructions clear and unambiguous?

The safe environment can be constructed both physically and psychologically. The former is dealt with here.

As discussed earlier in the chapter dealing with discussions, a small closed circle is ideal for open discussions. One variation of this seating arrangement is referred to as the "Goldfish bowl". This is shown in the Figure 5.1. The role play is initially carried out in the centre of the circle. Afterwards the participants rejoin the circle for the debriefing.

The arrangement of chairs in the centre can be used to facilitate different kinds of role play. For example, participants may be placed face to face for discussion, or back to back for simulated "faceless" telephone contact.

Scenarios

As mentioned above, scenarios are a form of improvised role play in which the clinical care of patients is practised. Preparation of the environment is not only essential for the scenario to succeed, it is probably the most important part of the set. The equipment, manikins, and models, the layout of the station, and the way in which the learners will fit into the environment all have to be planned. A simple checklist may help.

Equipment

It is essential that all the equipment that might be required during the treatment of a real patient is available for use during scenario teaching. Any deficiencies can best be noted by running through the expected course of care before the session. If deficiencies cannot be made up, then a decision should be taken about how particular items of equipment will be enacted. It is often better to decide to make a particular item "notional" rather than ask learners to imagine that one item of equipment is actually another.

Scenario participants frequently generate the same kind of emotional intensity experienced in role play and therefore it is important that all equipment is made safe. To this end, all real needles and sharp surgical instruments should be removed, and potentially dangerous items such as defibrillators and lasers should be either inactivated or reduced in power so that they are harmless. This is particularly important if live patient models are used.

Manikins or models?

Despite manikins being designed to be as realistic as possible for a given clinical situation, they are, of course, dolls, with the

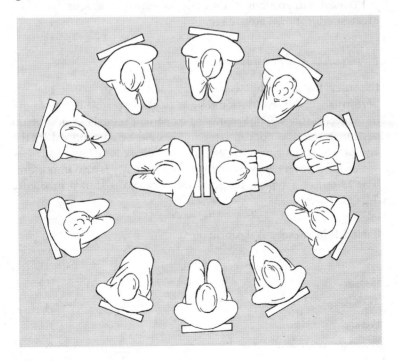

Figure 5.1   Goldfish bowl seating arrangement

41

disadvantage that they do not move. Learners have to suspend belief because of this basic flaw, and teachers must therefore provide the dynamic for the situation. To achieve this they must understand the strengths and weaknesses of the manikin, and must be completely *au fait* with the way in which it operates. Failure of the instructor to operate the manikin correctly will at best disrupt and at worst destroy the teaching session.

Patient models are able to provide real patient responses, although they must still be thoroughly briefed so that they understand the nature and course of their supposed condition. To allow learners to interact with them realistically they should be made up to appear ill, since most learners find an apparently well live patient model is even less believable than a manikin. Most procedures cannot be carried out on real models, therefore definite steps have to be taken to ensure their safety and to preserve their modesty.

The relative merits of manikins and live patient models are summarised in Table 5.1.

In most circumstances properly designed manikins have the greatest educational advantage.

Layout and learner interactions

In order to allow the learners to carry out or see a realistic performance, the layout should be as close as possible to that found in clinical settings. Thus manikins or patient models should be on beds or trolleys as appropriate, and should be surrounded by the equipment and fittings that would normally accompany this.

For the learners viewing the scenario visibility is also important. The layout of a typical resuscitation scenario is shown in Figure 5.2

Table 5.1: Manikins *v.* real patient models

	Manikin	Real patient model
Realism	+	+ +
Appearance	+	+ +
Verbal/physical interaction	+	+ +
Procedure performance	+ +	−
Safety	+ +	+

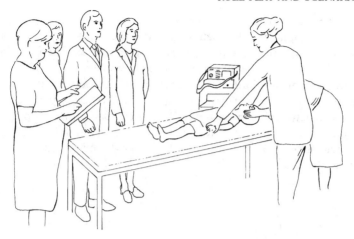

Figure 5.2   Layout of a typical resuscitation scenario

Set

Mood and motivation are particulary important during scenario teaching since learners are essentially being asked to suspend belief and to pretend to be involved in an imaginary situation. This is helped if the content and objectives of the whole session are rehearsed. The group taking part in the scenario should be briefed together. In addition, each individual should receive a separate briefing, either written or verbally. It is important to check before the scenario that all participants are happy with the parts they are to play.

In scenario teaching, it is particularly important to ensure that the learner who is to carry out the clinical intervention has fully understood the situation. To check this the learner should be asked to repeat the description of the scenario to the teacher before beginning.

Particular problems or peculiarities of the scenario (such as items of notional equipment, or how physiological variables will be indicated) should also form part of the set.

Dialogue

The dialogue during role play is interesting since the instructor is no longer in complete control. In prepared role play the teacher may predefine parameters within which the situation is confined.

In improvised role play teachers will have no control if they are not part of the play. In these circumstances the set must be used to define the nature of the play – it is, however, impossible to predict how the participants will perform until they start.

In scenario teaching, the teacher retains an active part in the session in that the learner or group of learners are dependent on the instructor for clinical input. This input can either be passive (learner-requested) or active (instructor-initiated). In either case the teacher can exert some control over the direction and outcome of the session.

Inform
  of clinical progress as requested
  of clinical changes which cannot be deduced

Listen
  to statements from the learners and act appropriately

Respond
  give physiological parameters not available from the equipment

---

In addition to providing the patient's physiological responses instructors can intervene to slow down/speed up the action as required. This may involve either verbal or physical interventions. The former will include prompting and/or questioning to draw out/move on. The latter may involve performing some action for the learner or some other action such as sitting down or pacing up and down.

The session should be TERMINATED IMMEDIATELY IF SAFETY IS COMPROMISED, for instance by dangerous use of instruments or defibrillators.

Debriefing

The importance of debriefing after a role play was emphasised earlier. Time must be allowed to enable participants to talk out their feelings and be guided back to normality by the instructor.

Closure

As with all types of teaching, role play and scenarios should be closed by allowing time for questions, by summarising the content of the session, and then by a clear termination.

There may be a number of questions outstanding at the end of this type of session since. As alluded to above, the content will be to some degree learner-driven. These should be answered as appropriate and as time allows. Questions that are peripheral to the overall aim of the session, and those which might confuse the whole group, are best dealt with outside the session itself.

Once questions have been dealt with, the lessons learnt should be summarised. Once again the student-driven nature of these situations means that teachers must draw together the various topics covered, and place them in the context of the overall learning objectives. Students should be told of any areas that have not yet been covered, and should be told when and where such topics will be covered.

It is important that a clear termination is given and that time constraints are observed. This may involve choosing a new candidate to practise for another run-through, telling candidates to go to another skill station or for a break. It must be clear, concise, and short.

Checklist for scenarios

Environment

- Fix layout
- Check lighting
- Adjust heating/ventilation
- Check equipment
- Brief assistant

Set

- Set mood
- Establish usefulness/relevance
- State learning objectives
- Clarify learner/teacher roles

Dialogue

- Brief candidate
- Allow candidate to ask questions
- Check candidate's understanding of the briefing
- Position participants
- Direct the scenario purposefully
- Respond positively to the candidate's treatment strategies
- Do not allow the candidate to become too stressed
- Allow the candidate the opportunity to achieve the set aim
- Provide a positive critique

Closure

- Invite questions and/or comments
- Summarise
- Terminate

Example: A teaching plan for scenarios

Environment

Layout

Check layout and access
Check visibility
Check lighting
Adjust heating/ventilation

Equipment

Check layout of equipment
Check manikins

Equipment list

Scenario manikin
Heartsim rhythm simulator
Defibrillator
Selection of Minijet drugs (adrenaline, atropine etc.)
Adult self-inflating bag (1600 ml) with reservoir and valve
Non-rebreathing valves
Selection of adult face masks – 2, 3, 4, 5
Laryngeal mask airways – 3, 4, 5
Selection of adult oral airways – 2, 3, 4, 5
Selection of nasal airways – 6, 6.5, 7
Laerdal pocket mask with one-way valve and O_2 inlet
Oxygen tubing
Laryngoscope with Macintosh blade (spare bulb and batteries)
Endotracheal tubes – 6 mm, 7 mm, 8 mm, 9 mm
Catheter mount
Bandage
Yankauer sucker
Syringe
Magill forceps
Introducers – malleable and gum elastic
Stethoscope
Torch
Suction tubing
Venflons 14 g, 16 g
Portex connector
Syringes – 2 ml, 5 ml

Minitrach
O_2 masks

Set

Introduction
Explain the usefulness of the session

> "During the next 30 minutes we will undertake two simulated resuscitations. This will allow you to put into practice all the knowledge and skills we have covered so far . . ."

Explain the general content and style

> "One of you will lead the resuscitation, while others will be employed as members of the team. For each scenario I will ask one of you to critique the performance."

State the specific objectives:

Airway	Assess
	Establish airway patency
	Oral endotracheal intubation
Breathing	Bag-and-mask with added O_2
	Continued ventilation with 100% O_2
Circulation	VF protocol
	EMD protocol
General	Safety
	Uninterrupted BLS except for defib

Expected therapy

For expected therapy refer to current protocols

Dialogue

Brief the candidate:

> "During the scenario, you will have an assistant who will assist, but not prompt you. She is a junior staff nurse who can carry out basic life support, cardiac compressions and bag-valve-mask ventilation if requested. During the scenario, I will give you any clinical signs you ask for."

48

Direct the scenario from the template given:

HISTORY
A 45 year-old-male suddenly loses consciousness.

Paramedic or GP – called to the scene by wife. You have a colleague with you who can perform CPR but has no further skills. The patient has collapsed without any preceding symptoms.

Nurse or doctor (emergency department) – brought into the resuscitation room by a non-paramedic crew. They had been called to the house by the patient's wife following an attack of chest pain. Patient lost consciousness in transit. The rest of the department is busy but you have a junior colleague who can perform CPR.

Nurse or doctor (ward) – admitted 4 hours previously to your ward following an anterior infarct. No previous history. Seemed to be doing well, aspirin had been given in the Emergency Department and streptokinase has been started. An IV line is in place and the patient is connected to a monitor. Initially the only assistant is a junior nurse who can perform CPR.

INITIAL OBSERVATIONS
Pulseless and apnoeic.

INSTRUCTOR'S INFORMATION

Diagnosis – Cardiorespiratory arrest following an anterior myocardial infarction.

Clinical course – The patient is initially in VF and remains in this rhythm until after the first three shocks and adrenaline have been given. Following a transient recovery, the patient develops a tension pneumothorax and a narrow complex sinus tachycardia. Eventually EMD ensues. If this is treated by needle thoracocentesis, the patient regains a palpable pulse but remains unconscious and requires ventilatory support. The monitor shows a heart rate of 90–100 with occasional VEs. Blood pressure is 100 mmHg. The patient requires ICU for post-resuscitation care.

Provide a critique

Closure

Ask if there are any questions
Summarise

> "In this session we have put together the knowledge and skills you have learnt elsewhere."

Terminate the session

6 Assessment

This chapter deals with the theory and practice of assessment. After reading it you should:

- **understand** the underlying principles of assessment
- **be aware** of the common methods of assessment
- **be able** to prepare a formal and informal assessment

Assessment enables teachers to determine whether the required standard of performance has been achieved by the learner. For an assessment to have any meaning it is essential that it has the following features:

- **Specificity**   it incorporates either a subjective or objective assessment of a defined feature
- **Validity**   it tests what it claims to test
- **Reliability**   the same result would be achieved with the same learner if the assessment was repeated with different examiners in a different place
- **Feasibility**   it does not require prohibitive resources
- **Fidelity**   it is an accurate reflection of real life

The design of assessments is always a compromise. Those that are tightly constructed with little room for subjective judgements will probably be more reliable but have less validity and fidelity. In contrast, subjective assessments are likely to be less reliable, but may be more valid and true to life. To overcome the latter problem, subjective assessments should incorporate some form of checklist, and should be conducted by at least two teachers.

It is relatively straightforward to define specific, objective criteria to determine the cognitive and psychomotor competence of candidates. For example, "Intubation must be correctly complete within 30 seconds". Such assessments are known as **criterion-referenced**. In contrast, defining criteria for attitudes and interpersonal relationships is notoriously difficult. Despite this difficulty, it may be important to carry out such assessments as people who have difficulties in relating to others or those with inappropriate attitudes can undermine a whole team.

Forms of assessment

Formal and informal assessments

Assessment of learners can take place in a formal situation or may occur informally. In the first case, both the learner and the teacher are aware of the assessment, which tends to be criterion-based. In the second situation often only the teacher is aware of the assessment, which is more subjective.

In many situations an informal assessment of learners' abilities in lectures, skill stations, discussion groups and in role plays/scenarios can be invaluable to both the teacher (to see whether the learners understand what is being taught) and to the learner (to understand whether they are progressing satisfactorily).

In some situations formative assessment may be formalised by the use of score sheets. Such sheets can also be used as a means of recording.

Final assessment is carried out at the testing stations which have been designed to assess knowledge ("must know" and "should know"), practical skills ("can show"), and the actual application of knowledge and practical skills in scenarios and role play.

Formative and summative assessments

Once a meaningful assessment has been developed and carried out, it is possible to inform the candidate how they are progressing during the course or teaching session. This is called **formative assessment** and it has an educational aim because it enables the teacher to guide and encourage the candidate. Conversely, **summative assessment** is carried out at the end of the educational episode and has an administrative aim in determining whether or not a satisfactory standard had been reached.

Any assessment may be either formal or informal and either formative or summative. The use of the various combinations is shown in Table 6.1. Care must be taken in making sure the right form of assessment is being used.

Table 6.1: Use of different assessments

	Formative	Summative
Formal	Initial test	Final criteria tests
Informal	Continuous subjective	Final subjective

Types of assessment

Knowledge

Knowledge that is required to complete a short course success-fully can be assessed by short answers. Multiple choice questions (MCQ) can also assess the basic level of knowledge quite well, but questions need careful design and must be trialled before regular use.

Psychomotor

Technical skills can be assessed using mechanical simulation or a manikin. Practical tests must be assessed for validity and reliability and, within the constraints of manikin design, fulfil the require-ment for fidelity to the actual clinical situation. It should be remembered that tests are rarely conducted in real clinical situations, and instructors therefore have a major part to play in achieving fidelity. Each station must be carefully set up with this in mind, and each candidate should be fully briefed before entering the testing area.

Social behaviour

Rather than carrying out criterion-referenced assessment of attitudes and interpersonnel relationships, informal assessment may be used. Informal assessments are made throughout the course in all contexts. Multiple assessments of each candidate will increase validity, eliminate bias and provide a comprehensive view of the candidate's abilities and enable those with instructor potential to be identified. These can then be assigned various teaching tasks so that this potential can be further assessed.

Critiquing enables candidates to demonstrate their knowledge of the subject as well as their ability to correct their colleagues' performances constructively. In doing so, the affective and inter-personal aspects of behaviour can be assessed.

Scenario

Scenario tests allow three aspects of learner behaviour to be assessed (knowledge, psychomotor skills and social behaviour). Instructor preparation and briefing of candidates for testing are vitally important if a test is to fulfil its purpose. Poor instructor preparation (such as failing to understand the scenario, failing to brief the assistant, and failing to learn how to operate the manikin) will reduce both the validity and fidelity of the test. Reliability is achieved by ensuring that all instructors operate a particular station in almost exactly the same way. Instructors should discuss the candidate performance and measure it against set critieria. Successful candidates will achieve the key points necessary for good care.

If it is clear within 5 minutes that a learner cannot achieve the standard then the test must be stopped, since little can be gained educationally from prolonging an irretrievable situation. In some situations it may be possible to restart the test immediately.

Learners should be informed of the result as soon as the test finishes. In cases where the result is in doubt, the candidate should be asked to wait outside the test area whilst the instructors discuss the case. Table 6.2 summarises the appropriate types of assessment.

Table 6.2: Assessment types

Knowledge	MCQ short answer questions
Psychomotor	Skills test
Knowledge Psychomotor Interpersonal/social	Scenario

Checklist for assessment

Environment

- Fix layout
- Check lighting
- Adjust heating/ventilation
- Check equipment is:
    working
    in place
- Brief assistant where appropriate

Set

- Brief candidate:
    clearly
    calmly
    set objectives
- Allow candidate to ask questions

Dialogue

- Give candidate the opportunity to achieve set aim
- Interact constructively

Closure

- Finish session positively
- Detect
    areas of strength
    areas of weakness
- Correctly detect pass/fail
- Inform candidate of result

Example: Criteria for testing

Basic airway

- Chin lift and jaw thrust
- Use of suction
- Sizing and insertion of oropharyngeal airway
- Sizing and insertion of nasopharyngeal airway
- Adequate ventilation of an adult manikin 3 times using pocket mask with supplemental oxygen
- Adequate ventilation of an adult manikin 3 times using a bag-valve-mask and a 1- or 2-person technique

Scenario

- Airway and cervical spine
  Assess
  Tracheal intubation
  Protect cervical spine

- Breathing
  High flow O_2
  Ventilation once intubated

- Circulation
  Assessment
  IV access $\times$ 2
  IV crystalloid or colloid boluses
  Blood transfusion
  Call surgeon

PART TWO

BACKGROUND
INFORMATION

7 Adult learning

This chapter is concerned with the special features of adults as learners. After reading it you should:

- **understand** how adults learn
- **be aware** of how to promote adult learning

This section looks in more detail at the adult status of learners and the implications of this for teaching. Learning can be defined as a "relatively permanent change in an individual's behaviour resulting from experience". In life we are exposed to a vast array of learning experiences, some of which are pleasant and some of which are not. Though we learn from bad experiences as much as from positive ones, the tendency is for painful experiences to promote either an avoidance or a defensive response. As neither of these actions will help the learners when they attempt to put theory into practice, this type of learning should be avoided.

Learners

Adult learners bring with them their own individual ways of working and each learner is unique. However, they also share certain characteristics which should be kept in mind by the trainer.

Needs

Adults learn best when the educational experience ensures that:

- The content is relevant and has meaning and purpose for everyday issues
- The learner is actively involved
- Objectives are defined and goals set
- Positive feedback is given
- Reflection on the learning experience is encouraged

Teachers of adults should adapt their teaching to accommodate these features. Relevance should be ensured by relating to the candidates' experiences, by asking candidates to apply new knowledge and skills to their everyd?·· working context and by suggesting possible applications.

Active participation should be encourag... ⅰ ⅰⅰⅰ꞉ can be achieved by conducting interactive lectures with opportunities for questioning, application and reflection. Skill stations, scenarios, workshops and discussions are participative and should be included in learning programmes for this reason.

Needs can be identified and goals set by negotiation with the learners. Not all candidates are clear about what they want or what they need to do to get it. The teacher's experience can be valuable here in helping to set realistic goals for individual candidates.

Positive feedback must be provided – through positive critiquing of performance and through the positive reception of candidates' contributions. Positive feedback also includes enabling individuals to identify their weakness and devising remedies.

Reflection can be encouraged – through summaries, during lecture activities and during mentor time, candidates' learning is enhanced by reflection.

Variations

There are important variations between the individuals who attend your courses. These include differences in, for instance, past experiences, future needs, specialisms and, of course, motivation and ability. These will result in a variety of abilities. The learners may have had previous training, good or bad, or have been exposed to situations they felt ill-prepared to cope with. As a result of these factors and many more, a whole spectrum of requirements for these learners will exist. All these aspects should be taken into account when a session is being planned.

8 The domains of learning

This chapter is concerned with the four domains of learning. After reading it you should:

- **understand** that learning takes place in stages
- **be aware** of the stages within the four domains of learning

Learning can be classified into four main areas or domains, these are:

- Knowledge
- Skills
- Attitudes
- Relationships

When we consider "learning" we tend to think of knowledge and its recall and the performance of psychomotor skills. Few think of attitudes (such as being considerate, responsible, arrogant or patronising) or of social relationships (such as being able to communicate, delegate or lead) as part of learning. However, attitudes and relationships are as important as knowledge and skill in the promotion of effective performance.

Each of these four domains can be further broken down into stages of learning. They are dealt with in turn below.

Knowledge

Our knowledge increases gradually as with experience, reflection, and further study we come to appreciate the complexity of issues. Knowledge is acquired in six stages, which are:

- Knowledge
- Comprehension
- Application
- Analysis
- Synthesis
- Evaluation

The most basic level of cognitive learning entails a straight recollection of facts and is called **knowledge** – for example, the learner may know the correct intravenous dose of adrenaline. In certain situations this kind of knowledge is adequate, but to use a drug appropriately it is also necessary to be familiar with both indications for use and contraindications. Clearly this is a higher level of learning and it is known as **comprehension**. This allows the use of the drug in different situations.

The **application** level is reached when the learner relies upon his/her knowledge of an intervention to use it correctly in a real or simulated situation. During this active phase the next level of learning also occurs; this is called **analysis** and results from the learner attempting to "observe" the effect of an intervention in the light of his/her prior knowledge.

As a consequence of this analysis, a new level of understanding of the intervention is reached and its actions can be related to outcome by a process known as **synthesis**. This ultimate level of learning is called **evaluation** when the whole process and its results are reflected upon and judged. The outcomes of this judgement will determine the next course of action and the quality of the learning which has occurred.

Skills

The learning of practical, psychomotor skills depends on the coordination between the brain and the motor and sensory systems. There are four stages involved:

- Perception
- Guided response
- Mastery
- Autonomy

During **perception** the learner becomes aware of the skill and begins to appreciate some of the movements required to perform the skill, as well as the potential difficulties involved. Often the skill is mentally broken down by the learner in anticipation of the next stage, where initial performance takes place. Perception is the basis for stages 1 and 2 of the four-stage method of teaching skills. During the **guided response** the learner is actively engaged in working through the skill either verbally (stage 3) or physically (stage 4). At the end of stage 4 learners should have acquired the technique but they will not be "skilled". With practice they should reach the **mastery** stage when they can perform the skill competently (as one might drive a car when passing the driving test). With further practice the **autonomy** stage should be reached. At this level the skill itself can be performed with little conscious thought (as one no longer needs to think about clutch, accelerator or brake when driving). Instead concentration can be focused elsewhere, such as on the total wellbeing of the patient or the activities of the team (or on safely navigating through traffic rather than thinking about the mechanical aspects of driving).

Mastery or autonomy will seldom be achieved during short courses because of time constraints. It is important to advise learners that any new techniques must be assessed critically to ensure appropriateness and safety.

Attitudes

The learning of attitudes also has four stages, which are:

• Perceiving
• Complying
• Accepting
• Internalising

Perceiving requires the learner to recognise an issue towards which an attitude might be formed. As examples, issues such as feminism, ethnicity, sexual orientation, and political correctness have emerged over the past 30 years or so. At some stage everyone becomes aware for the first time that these are of sufficient importance to merit thought.

Learners, however, cannot be allowed the luxury of gradually realising that certain attitudes are important. Areas such as safety, teamwork or sensitivity to relatives need to be addressed directly – all in the context of the knowledge and skills they will support.

Unfortunately, there is no guarantee that simply telling a learner a particular attitude is important will ensure that they adopt the ethic. Learners are actually quite likely to appear to **comply** with the instructor whether they agree or not. Continued exposure to **consistent** teaching, and the subsequent testing of attitudes in real environments, may well bring the learner to **accept** the values taught. At this stage the learner has come to see that such values may be important in real situations. The final stage is reached when reservations are dropped and the learner recognises these attitudes as being of value in their own right –the learner then **internalises** the attitudes and makes them his or hers, they become part of the person, expressed in all contexts not only the educational one.

Relationships

In many situations actual interventions are carried out by teams rather than individuals. Within the team individuals will have differing expertise. The group's dynamics and ability to carry out its designated tasks is dependent upon the interpersonal skills of the team members. The key elements of these are:

- **Decisions**   Friendly/unfriendly
- **Tension**   Agreeing/disagreeing
- **Reintegration**   Providing support

- **Communication**   Asking for and giving information
- **Control**   Asking for and giving opinions
- **Evaluation**   Asking for and giving guidance

All the features listed above are present in a creative group. However, the key to success is the group's ability to resolve tensions and disagreements. This requires a variety of roles: e.g. the timekeeper, the gatekeeper on information, the ideas person, the facilitator. However, these roles are not fixed. Commonly in any group members will play different roles at different times. In this way the group can develop cognitive and psychomotor skills together.

9 Giving feedback

This chapter is concerned with giving feedback. After reading it you should:

- **understand** the role of feedback in the educational experience
- **be aware** of the importance of positive feedback.

Giving feedback is a core skill for any teacher. The kind and quality of feedback, when it is given, and the way in which it is given are all highly significant for the learning process and for learner motivation. Feedback, whether given formally during a critique, or given informally through nods and smiles, tells the learner how they are progressing towards their goal of acquiring knowledge or mastering a skill.

Unfortunately, there are some cultural hurdles to overcome in order to give good feedback. Having watched a performance, especially one in an area where we are relatively expert, our cultural inclination is to say what was wrong with it – thus demonstrating our own expertise. But for most performances the "wrong" part, the inadequate part, constitutes a small proportion of the whole. Most of it was good but we neglect to tell the performer this in favour of concentrating on the inadequate. Learners, of course, share this culture and will want to defend themselves, forestalling criticism by informing their observers that they are well aware of all the inadequacies of their performance. They will be reluctant to admit to any aspect of it being acceptable let alone good. Against these cultural expectations the teacher has to give feedback which is **accurate** and will assist the learner in **making progress** with their learning. The scheme outlined below will achieve this.

- Ask the learner what went well in their performance/presentation, or what they were particularly pleased with.
- Ask the group what they felt went well. When they have finished, add your own observations about what went well.

- Ask the learner what, if they were to repeat the performance, they would wish to improve upon.
- Ask the group what suggestions they have which would improve the performance. When they have finished, add your own suggestions.
- Summarise the good points and the main suggestions for improvement.

There are a number of points at which this process can be undermined. Learners will not want to say what they felt went well with their performance. When asked they will typically say – "Nothing really, I didn't do . . ." At this point it is necessary to intervene and insist that they identify something good within the performance. The group may begin by identifying good points and then drift off into – "But I didn't really like the way you . . ." They have to be reminded here that you are dealing with the good points. Again when asking the group for suggestions for improvement some will still want to say what was "wrong", for example, "You didn't handle your overheads very well", whereas what is needed are suggestions for improvement such as, "If you put your overheads on the left hand side and then on the chair after use the changeovers would work much more smoothly". Finally, too many suggestions for improvement will only confirm the learner's sense of inadequacy and would be practically impossible to implement hence the need to prioritise the feedback given.

The term positive feedback may, at times, give the wrong impression. At worst it may be taken to mean that only "nice" things may be said. It is positive because it helps the learner improve. Learners cannot improve unless they know **where** improvement is necessary and **how** the improvements may be made. This is positive feedback. Identifying the "where" without the "how" is negative feedback which informs the learners of their inadequacies but offers no remedial help.

10 Asking questions

This chapter is concerned with questions and questioning techniques. After reading it you should:

- **understand** the role of questioning and how to respond to answers
- **be aware** of the levels at which questions can be asked

Questions are an integral part of teaching because:

- They allow the teacher to relate directly to the learner(s)
- They provide the teacher with feedback
- They enable the learners to be active and to participate
- They can require the learner to articulate views and to share understandings
- They can require the individuals to reflect on and relate to practice

Questions reflect the six stages of knowledge discussed in Chapter 8.

The instructor needs to decide what kinds of questions will be appropriate to a particular session and to be clear about their purposes. Questions from too high a stage of knowledge will frighten and alienate learners if used too soon; also those from too low a stage may patronise.

Time availability is a major factor which must be taken into account when deciding upon the level of question to be asked. Lower level questions tend to generate single word answers, whereas higher levels can give rise to discussion or debate. Consequently, lower level questions are commonly used in lectures and practical sessions where quick repetition of data is required. In contrast, higher level questions tend to be used in group discussion work.

The stages of knowledge are:

- Knowing
- Understanding
- Applying/Analysing
- Synthesising
- Evaluating

The level of a question is set by the words used in this construction. Each level is defined below, and suitable examples are given.

Knowledge

Identify, state, name, tell, write, define, tick, list, describe.

Do you remember, who, when, what, where, how many, which, how big/wide/much, does?

Comprehension

Compare, distinguish, show, find the evidence, try to prove, interpret, re-arrange, re-state, explain the difference, organise.

Which are alike, what do you infer, how are these common, what is different?

Application/analysis

Specify conditions for, arrange, demonstrate, make use of, illustrate/give an example of, explore, discover, form a hypothesis.

What are the consequences, what conclusion, what is necessary, under what circumstances, how can you use it, what are the problems, what are the causes, how could you?

Synthesis

Solve this, think of a new approach, create, devise, speculate, imagine, design.

What do you suggest, if . . . changes what alternatives are there, how many different ways, what would happen if?

Evaluation

Check the results to prove the point, evaluate this set of data against the standards, rate order of preference, according to your understanding, according to what happened, argue all sides.

How do you rate it, what do you think will succeed, why, which, is there a better solution, is it good/bad, was it right/wrong, will it work?

For questions to be most effective they must be planned prior to the teaching session. Furthermore, instructors should practise using their bodies and voices so that questions do not come over as too threatening. Finally, once an answer is received, teachers need to deal with them. These may be right, wrong or not forthcoming, but each response must be dealt with appropriately.

What the tutor can get wrong

Discussions will function less effectively when the tutor:

- Asks ambiguous or confusing questions
- Asks more than one question at once
- Asks a question and answers it him/herself
- Fails to listen to what the participants say or ignores their answers
- Fails to see the implications of answers for developing issues and points
- Fails to develop (or facilitate development of) answers
- Uses the discussion to give a lecture or to tell anecdotes

11 Handling difficult learners

This chapter is concerned with the recognition and handling of difficult learners. After reading it you should:

- **understand** the types of difficult learners
- **be aware** of the various strategies for handling them

As discussed earlier, most adult learners are highly motivated and enthusiastic participants in well-designed educational scenarios. Sometimes, however, individual learners can cause teachers difficulties. For the sake of clarity these have been divided into three types:

- Talkers
- Non-talkers
- Destroyers

Talkers

These learners are usually extremely enthusiastic and want to show the instructor that they have a sound core knowledge. As such they tend to monopolise the discussion. Unfortunately, this can have an extremely negative effect on group dynamics, and may prevent any form of group discussion. Teachers should, therefore, be aware of techniques that can be used to influence this type of candidate.

One approach is for the instructor to summarise, or ask the candidate to summarise, what has been said. This allows the candidate's comments to be used positively. Following the summary the focus of the discussion can be directed to another member of the group. This technique can be used for candidates who talk too quickly. It is important to use learners' comments constructively. Occasionally, when enthusiasm gets the better of a participant the topic of discussion may deviate from what is expected. Again, micro-summaries are useful to recapitulate and then redirect the discussion.

It is often very difficult to interject while learners like these are talking. To overcome this teachers should wait until the talker has to breathe, then thank them for their response, rephrase it, and redirect the discussion.

Occasionally in a discussion group, one or two learners may engage in a satellite discussion which may or may not be related to the topic in question. Irrespective of this, it is still a disrupting influence. To cope with this the teacher may stop the main discussion, listen to the satellite one, and link this with the main discussion and thereby reamalgamate the group. Alternatively, a direct approach such as calling the particular talker by name can be used to draw them back into the discussion.

Non-talkers

"Non-talker" does not necessarily equate to "non-learner", but having said this some candidates who do not actively participate in discussions may need a tremendous amount of support.

Nervous candidates must be given encouragement. On questioning they may respond with totally inappropriate answers. Teachers should avoid negative, derogatory, or destructive responses. Redirection or rephrasing of the initial question can be employed to avoid embarrassment of the candidate in front of their peers. It is up to the teacher to control the situation and, for example, say "Sorry, I did not phrase that particularly well", and then rephrase the question so that the candidate's response is more acceptable. Repeating or summarising the candidate's ideas may make them feel more comfortable. Learners feel most comfortable in familiar situations. This can be exploited by placing questions in the usual context – for example, the question "As a coronary care charge nurse I am sure that you have seen many patients with atrial flutter. What problems have you encountered in treating this condition?" may well allow a nervous candidate from a coronary care unit to collect their thoughts and express them.

Destroyers

Unfortunately learners who fall into this category often have a negative attitude and can be extremely destructive to the group. They may appear aloof because they know that they understand the core knowledge and feel reluctant to share this knowledge with others. Despite the temptation to do otherwise, it is important that the instructor should attempt to help these learners use their knowledge constructively, pointing out how they can help others to learn.

Obstinate candidates may either fail to see the point during the discussion or remain completely prejudiced by their previous knowledge and fail to accept or even acknowledge the group's opinion. In such circumstances learners' peers should be encouraged to try to influence this isolated opinion and, hence, draw an obstinate candidate into the group.

With the candidate who is complaining it is important to establish whether the complaint is legitimate or not. If the complaint is minor, the situation should be rectified immediately and the group's attention refocused on the discussion. Major complaints may need to be resolved away from the group. If possible a constructive attitude should be maintained – comments can be used, expanded upon, and used to involve the remainder of the group.

Occasionally, candidates are argumentative, rude, and resistant to manipulative techniques. Under these circumstances it is advisable to try to engage the individual concerned in private. If the candidate's attitude is not amenable to change, and he/she is at risk of disrupting the whole learning experience, then the possibility that a "personality clash" has precipitated the candidate's grievances must be considered. Another teacher should discuss the situation with the learner. In the unlikely event that the situation cannot be rectified at all, the candidate should be asked to leave.

12 Beyond teaching

This chapter is concerned with the individual and group responsibilities of instructors above and beyond that of teaching. After reading it you should:

- **understand** the additional roles of teachers beyond teaching
- **be aware** of how these roles can be fulfilled

Attending meetings

On many organised courses there are teachers' meetings (faculty meetings) at the beginning of the course and at the end of each day. The initial meeting is a forum for all teachers to meet since often they may not know each other and have probably not all taught together before. The course director and the course coordinator can introduce instructors to each other, discuss the layout of the teaching environment, note any last minute changes to the programme, and importantly, discuss the approach to any contentious areas that are being addressed.

The initial meeting also provides an opportunity to ensure that all teachers are prepared for the day ahead. Instructors teaching overlapping topics can use the opportunity to check which areas they are each covering and to ensure a consistent approach.

Instructors' meetings at the end of the day should be more focused on the candidates themselves, although any logistical or controversial issues which have arisen during the day will be discussed and rectified. The main aim of a discussion of candidates is to identify those who need remedial help and to formulate a plan to deliver this. The assessments which are collated from any formative feedback sheets should be used to assist in this process.

At the final instructors' meeting any formative and summative assessments are discussed. On some courses learners may pass, retest in a particular area or it may be recommended that they repeat the course in its entirety. Some participants may be offered the opportunity to teach.

Supporting learners

Many structured courses involve learners taking an intensive training programme, in a format which they have often not experienced before. Teachers need to help the learners by providing a link and a support throughout. This is often called mentoring.

An instructor who is acting as a mentor should make early contact with the learner and make arrangements to maintain regular contact throughout the course. Learners may only need reassurance that they are progressing well, may need support in the form of brief remedial teaching sessions, or may require considerable input around areas they are concerned about.

The mentor will:

• Attempt to develop individual learners' potential
• Enable individual learners to identify their abilities and inabilities
• Identify possible remedial action
• Assist individual learners to make informed decisions on the direction of their development

Mentors will need to take any opportunity to observe and to talk to the learners and in so doing should become aware of any special abilities they may have. These abilities may include expertise with equipment, knowledge of topics and capacity for relating easily to others. Mentors may also become aware of individual learner weaknesses and the areas where they need additional help. Even though such areas may be obvious to the mentor and perhaps the rest of the group, they may be far less obvious to the learner. In this case it may be necessary to spend some time counselling the learner– asking whether the performance was satisfactory and assessing how it might be improved. Ideally, the learners themselves should reach realistic judgements about their abilities and their inabilities. The mentor should then be able to outline possible courses of action to further develop particular talents or to remedy inadequacies.

The mentor/individual learner relationship will be:

- supportive
- based on trust
- non-judgemental
- non-directive
- honest

Only solutions initiated by the learner stand any chance of success. Therefore the mentor's task is to help them work through any problems to identify possible solutions, and to understand the consequences of the choices to be made. This becomes most difficult where performance is poor and where failing the course is a possibility. Telling candidates that they are failing to achieve pass levels is more likely to promote rejection than if they reach those conclusions for themselves. Being supportive does not preclude being honest and in the end the candidate must have a clear picture of his/her abilities.

One of the ways of developing a more systematic approach to mentoring is provided by an adaptation of Maslow's hierarchy of needs. Maslow argued that only when we have satisfied our most basic needs can we move onto our higher needs. Table 12.1

Table 12.1: Maslow's hierarchy of needs and the mentor role

Maslow's hierarchy	Mentor–learner interaction
Physiological needs	Has the candidate had enough sleep, rest or food? Has he/she had a particularly long journey or is he/she suffering from stress?
Security needs	Does the candidate feel confident in passing opinions, in attempting new skills, in asking questions, in admitting to not knowing?
Belonging needs	Does the candidate feel accepted by the group and by faculty?
Esteem needs	Does the candidate feel confident in his/her own abilities and is he/she aware that these competencies are valued by others?
Cognitive needs	Does the candidate understand the content of the course? Is he/she mastering the concepts involved?
Self-actualisation	Is the candidate's potential being maximised? Does the candidate feel satisfied with his/her development/progress?

expands on this and is intended to stimulate thought and identify possibilities rather than present a list of solutions.

The role of the mentor is not always straightforward. The opportunities for contact are often short and time is precious. Teachers may also have to prepare for future sessions, eat, and fulfil other roles. This can mean that mentoring is often rushed; the real skill of a mentor is to identify those candidates who can cope with this, and those who really do need more support. Sometimes other tasks will have to be passed on to other instructors.

Supporting Other Teachers

Occasionally, the teacher who is carrying out a session is less confident and may require both moral and actual support. Instructors must show support for teachers in this position both by "being there" (for instance, by sitting in at the back of the lecture room) and by stepping in to answer difficult questions raised by candidates.

Feeding Back

The quality of the educational experience for learners depends both on the standard of teaching and on the materials used to deliver it. Many courses are supported by comprehensive teaching packages. Instructors are the "front-line" users of these materials. As such they often notice problems with either the teaching package or process that have not been anticipated. It is important that these problems are fed back. Most packages are under constant review by Working Groups and are revised every 2–4 years. Teachers are in a good position to play an active role in this process.

Regulations and Requirements

Each governing body has similar, but slightly differing regulations with regard to completing instructor candidacies, maintaining instructor status, and recertification and it is important to familiarise yourself with these early on.

Governing bodies maintain central lists of all qualified instructors, and these are made available to course centres to allow them to invite instructors to teach. Instructors will also be sent lists of the course centres and course dates to allow them to approach suitable centres if they so wish.

APPENDIX

REFLECTIVE DIARY

Space is given here for a reflective diary for teachers. You should take the opportunity to fill in whatever you experience thus far, so that it can form the basis of discussions with fellow teachers and other mentors.

Good/bad teaching

What are the factors that indicate good or bad teaching?

Good Teaching	Bad Teaching

Lecturing

My Strengths	My Weaknesses

Skills teaching

My Strengths	My Weaknesses

Discussion groups

My Strengths	My Weaknesses

Role play

My Strengths	My Weaknesses

Notes

Notes

Notes

Notes

INDEX